Souping

The New Juicing - Detox, Cleanse & Weight Loss

Susie Campbell

Souping

© Copyright 2016 by Susie Campbell

All rights reserved.

In no way is it legal to reproduce, duplicate, or transmit any part of this document in either electronic means or in printed format. Recording of this publication is strictly prohibited and any storage of this document is not allowed unless with written permission from the publisher. All rights reserved.

The information provided herein is stated to be truthful and consistent, in that any liability, in terms of inattention or otherwise, by any usage or abuse of any policies, processes, or directions contained within is the solitary and utter responsibility of the recipient reader. Under no circumstances will any legal responsibility or blame be held against the publisher for any reparation, damages, or monetary loss due to the information herein, either directly or indirectly.
Respective authors own all copyrights not held by the publisher.

Legal Notice:
This book is copyright protected. This is only for personal use. You cannot amend, distribute, sell, use, quote or paraphrase any part or the content within this book without the consent of the author or copyright owner. Legal action will be pursued if this is breached.

Disclaimer Notice:
Please note the information contained within this document is for educational and entertainment purposes only. Every attempt has been made to provide accurate, up to date and

reliable complete information. No warranties of any kind are expressed or implied. Readers acknowledge that the author is not engaging in the rendering of legal, financial, medical or professional advice.

By reading this document, the reader agrees that under no circumstances are we responsible for any losses, direct or indirect, which are incurred as a result of the use of information contained within this document, including, but not limited to, —errors, omissions, or inaccuracies.

INTRODUCTION..7

CHAPTER ONE – SOUPING: MORE APPEALING THAN JUICING...10

WHAT IS SOUPING?..11
How does it work?..11
REASONS WHY SOUPING IS THE NEW JUICING..................................11
Souping has less sugar than juicing..11
Souping needs no special equipment..12
Soup is so easy to store..12
Souping is mentally less challenging to sustain than juicing..........12
Soups are loaded with a variety of veggies..................................13
Soup allows a benefit of the addition of a variety of herbs, spices, and broth..13
Juice limits the flavor diversity..13
MORE BENEFITS FROM SOUPING..14
It won't leave you feeling hungry..14
More textures..14
A FINAL WORD..15

CHAPTER TWO - CLEANSING AND DETOXIFYING YOUR BODY..16

WHAT IS BODY CLEANSING?..16
DETOXIFICATION HISTORY..16
WHY DO I NEED TO CLEANSE?..17
TYPES OF CLEANSING..17
Body/Organ Cleanses Versus Liquid Cleanses..................................17
Water Detox..18
Juice Cleanse/Detox..18
Master Cleanse..18
Milk Fasting..19
Beer Fasting..20
Soup Detox or 'Souping'..20
BENEFITS AND DISADVANTAGES TO CLEANSES, DETOXES, AND FASTS......20
Souping Versus Juice Detox..21
Juicing Advantages and Disadvantages..................................21

Susie Campbell

MEDICAL PROFESSIONALS QUESTION NECESSITY OF CLEANSING/DETOX..22

CHAPTER THREE – RECIPES...23
CREAMY VEGAN CAULIFLOWER SOUP W/ KALE GARLIC DRIZZLE............23
CREAMY TOMATO SOUP WITH BASIL..25
BEANS AND GREENS DETOX SOUP..28
DIET CABBAGE SOUP..31
DIET BEETROOT SOUP..33
COTTAGE CHEESE AND KALE SOUP..35
DIET LENTILS SOUP..39
GINGER AND BUTTERNUT SQUASH SOUP..40
RED PEPPER AND EDAMAME SOUP..43
VIETNAMESE TOFU NOODLE SOUP WITH BOK CHOY..............................45
MUSHROOM SOUP..48
ANTIQUE GRAINS SOUP...50
BLACK BEAN SOUP..51
RED LENTIL, SWEET POTATO AND COCONUT SOUP................................54
WATERCRESS SOUP..56
TOFU AND VEGETABLE SOUP..57
PUMPKIN AND GINGER SOUP..60
SPINACH AND TORTELLINI SOUP...61
TOFU AND VEGETABLE SOUP..62
SUMMERY PEA SOUP WITH TURMERIC SCALLOPS..................................65
TORTELLINI IN BRODO..67
TIMELESS MINESTRONE...69
CREAM OF MUSHROOM SOUP..71
BAKED POTATO SOUP...74
CREAM OF BROCCOLI SOUP..75
CAPRESE SOUP..78
CALDO VERDE...79
CELERIAC SOUP...80
HOT PARSNIP AND LENTIL SOUP WITH TRUFFLE OIL.............................83
BROCCOLI SOUP...84
SUPER NOODLE RAMEN WITH KALE AND BBQ MUSHROOMS...................85
PASTA E FAGIOLI SOUP...87
EASY AND DELICIOUS MISO SOUP..89
TURKEY AND COCONUT MILK SOUP...91
COLD CUCUMBER SOUP...94
TRADITIONAL GOULASH SOUP..95

Souping

CREAMY TOMATO BASIL SOUP..97
CREAMY CARROT SOUP WITH OATS...99
CREAMY CAULIFLOWER SOUP WITH KALE DRIZZLE................102
MISO SOUP..105
WHITE BEAN SOUP..108
SPICY CHICKEN TORTILLA SOUP...110
PIZZA SOUP..112
THAI LAKSA SOUP...115
POTATO SOUP.. 119
APPLE SQUASH SOUP... 122

CONCLUSION..125

Susie Campbell

Introduction

The juice cleanse has long been in the mainstream of modern health food, growing in bounds from its previous place in the secret caches of health gurus and yogis. These days everyone is aware of the virtues of fresh fruits and vegetables and the irreplaceable anti-oxidants they can supply. Even the corner gas station is today's supplier of fresh-pressed juices.

But now a new craze is quickly obsessing with the health virtuosos of America! The concept of souping is pretty basic — instead of consuming versions of the kale and carrot and beet recipes, some 'soupy' additions are thrown into the mix, like chicken broth and broccoli puree. However, the entire 'souping' enterprise still 'boils down' to a basic liquid diet.

And of course the marketing behind it preaches nourishment and not deprivation. Instead of using plastic or glass bottles of juice, many of the soups are presented in appealing bowls and perhaps decorated with an attractive organic garnish. And the soups can be served hot or cold and can tout their organic ingredients. And instead of losing the vegetable pulp or the fiber you're getting the entire vegetable.

Also it ends up being much more cost effective since there is no necessity to buy expensive and up-to-date juicers with all the bells and whistles. Another appeal of souping is the multitude of recipes available on the Internet or recipe books that can be replaced with organic veggies and fresh vegetable juices.

Souping

Five days of soup sounds more do-able and attractive than guzzling down green liquid kale and cauliflower for the same amount of time. But for folks who undoubtedly screw up their faces at the mere thought of drinking your vegetables but find warm savory soup to be infinitely more appealing plus still get the benefit of the cleanse, the appeal of souping seems to make a lot of sense.

When you decide to heal yourself via juicing- hunger is a daily shadow and no matter how many jars of kale and carrot you end up consuming. And your uncomfortable stomach will torture you with its rumblings. It is used to nourishment in the form of solid foot so, in this way, souping introduces some actual bulk into the mix including actual fiber and protein that should put a curb on that appetite for hours. If you have managed, in the past, to survive a five-day juice cleanse, souping may seem like a veritable breeze.

Winter invites the right feel for souping, as the thought of warmth from a bowl is very appealing. The brusque weather already dictates to our psyche to eat warm, comforting foods so the thought of making thick stews into thick and colorful bisques is not a stretch. In actual fact, the deliciousness of the cleanse definitely lessens the sacrifice and some people may actually look forward to it. Not many people will rush to do something if it is not appealing.

But the variety of soups now available from every day to the more exotic ones like curried lentil and kale, wild mushroom bisque and Moroccan chickpea and tomato might not sound like something that you'd look forward to on a "cheat day" but they are superbly alluring in themselves. Plus, when you actually make the soup at home you can incorporate the flavors of your personal tastes, not to mention individual and flavor-inducing spices and therefore, customize the end product to your liking.

And more to the point is the undeniable fact that getting more vegetables into the diet is a super way to get a power punch of nutrients and antioxidants that you probably would never get otherwise. Plus the fact that Flu season is still here and those germs are on the lookout for any run-down soul with low resistance, it is of superb wisdom to probably get a little more vitamin C and manganese, B vitamins, magnesium, etc. from all the vegetables. But keep in mind that souping is simply being used as a cleanse when it is incorporated singly into the diet. It is also a darn wonderful unit of gourmet food when eaten before a meal or with other food as well.

Chapter One

Souping: More Appealing than Juicing

Just eating better is actually a viable alternative to depriving oneself of bulk and fiber, as it is in actual juicing. It's not our natural inclination to drink our meals, no matter how healthy the juice concoction is. As a quick cleanse it works well but the recipient quickly loses interest and goes into a "When will this be done? -Mode."

The truth is that if we eat a veggie-loaded, well-combined diet on a regular, daily basis and at the right times with no late night binges or bags of cookies, our bodies will be able to actually go through its own natural cleanse without all the liquid.

To accelerate from eating no or very little vegetables to eating a load of them is almost a natural cleanse on its own. That is a good first step. Fine tuning it to eating so much more vegetables as you incorporate other healthy habits, raises the bar to a cleanse.

It has been said that everyone needs to detox and rest their body occasionally, but the select few who always eat a balanced diet, high in organic fruits and vegetables, devoid of excess sugar and fats, necessitate minimum detoxification

Proper souping is a less intensive, less extreme method of detoxifying our well-worked bodies.

What is souping?

Souping is a satisfying and delicious way to cleanse and infuse your body with tons of nutrients without the cold, impersonal method of drinking down cold juices.

How does it work?
Simple. Just make some batches of veggie-loaded soups and eat only these soups for a period of a few days. This allows your body to rest and get rid of toxins. It should also add notable energy to your step as you go.

Reasons Why Souping is the New Juicing

Souping is more cost efficient. Have you ever found yourself paying $60 at the Organic Food counter only to be able produce a few glasses of green goddess homemade juice; you will understand the high cost of juicing. And then just to toss all that pulp? It can be almost heart breaking. Soups are remarkably more inexpensive with absolutely no waste.

Souping has less sugar than juicing.
During the juicing process, the natural sugars of the fruit or vegetable will become concentrated in the juice whereas there is much less natural sugar in vegetables and that sugar will stay with the fiber which will reduce the amount you are absorbing.

Souping needs no special equipment.
There is no need to have to purchase an expensive juicer with all the components and features- you just need a large saucepan with a lid.

Soup is so easy to store.
An added benefit comes in the fact that you can easily store your homemade soups in the refrigerator for up to four or five days and up to 4-6 months in the freezer making the whole venture more sustainable.

Souping retains the fiber of the vegetable. When you don't have to throw out the bulk of the vegetable as you do with the pulp of the fruit you hold on to a good part of the fiber. So, not only providing your body with a wide variety of nutrients and minerals, souping retains the fiber and the integrity of the vegetable. And don't forget that you can add barley, quinoa, brown rice and fiber rich potatoes to the mix to add even more fiber.

And since fiber supports detoxification, that fact is a very good thing. Soluble fiber will aid and promote successful movement of the feces through the intestines and colon, as it binds many of the toxins in the bowel. This improves elimination.

Souping is mentally less challenging to sustain than juicing.
Because souping is more appealing it becomes more natural for the person doing the cleanse to participate. Souping is also kinder to your body and your mind. Naturally, it takes a bit of time for foods to travel to our stomachs and for our psyches to register that sensation of fullness. Juices are ingested quickly and take hardly any time to travel through the digestive system so rarely do you get that full feeling

from juicing. Thicker more concentrated food takes a good deal more time to digest. It can be critical to weight management, as well, to experience that sensation of fullness. It also leads to better assimilation of nutrients from the food.

It's also wise to give your body a little break for a few days or a week just consuming soups and provides a variety of vegetables that perhaps you have never had before or in such combination or amount.

Soups are loaded with a variety of veggies.
Juicing allows you to pack more servings of vegetables into one single meal but soups provide the same benefit while adding a wide variety of diverse vegetables to be consumed. Vegetables and many legumes like beans, root veggies and green leafy vegetables can be easily pureed in a blender. They not only provide increased energy and all the antioxidants you need, but they stabilize blood sugar as well.

Soup allows a benefit of the addition of a variety of herbs, spices, and broth.
Juicing uses fruits and sugars to create flavor and variety, but there are so many herbs and spices, as well as broths you can use to customize your soup.

Juice limits the flavor diversity.
Since juices are basically sweet by nature, they become limiting in the amount of flavors we can incorporate; ginger, parsley, mint and cinnamon and any sweet-complimenting taste is all that can be done. Souping lends itself to a whole new world of savory flavors, such as cumin, turmeric, pepper, cayenne, coriander, lemon, citrus, etc. to flavor the dish.

More Benefits from Souping

Herbs, spices and vegetables are rich in phytonutrients, which are nutrients inherent in vegetables and plants and possess an array of other active ingredients that are associated with the prevention and treatment of many common illnesses, conditions and disorders. These include cancer, diabetes, Alzheimer's, high blood pressure, and cholesterol and even chronic skin diseases like psoriasis and eczema.

You can literally also boost a soup's nutritional power in an instant! By using bone broth, or adding a scoop of miso (be doubly sure the soup isn't too hot when adding), or stirring in some chopped greens like, a bit of parsley, kale, chopped spinach, finely chopped Swiss chard, dandelion, beet greens or collards.

It won't leave you feeling hungry.
The extra bulk and fiber in soup, along with the soothing warmth will stay with you and not leave you wanting more food. Raw foods are actually more difficult to digest than food that is cooked. With souping, not only are you cooking the foods, but also the combination of more fiber and protein has staying power to keep you satisfied longer.

More textures.
Juice can get a bit mundane as you get tired of just drinking your meals. The variety of textures can help so much in keeping you interested longer. So if we can get all the benefits of cleansing through a more satisfying, flavorful and comforting means then why not?

A Final Word

Souping is a 'soup-er' project to start now in the cooler weather but it really does work year round. Look at different recipes and start to enjoy the soothing warmth of soups as well as their detoxifying effects soon. Start by making a variety of soups so you can choose the ones you love the best and you can be on the receiving end of all that nutrition.

A soup cleanse is not as difficult as you think as it does taste great and is not difficult to do. Just write down some of your favorite recipes and look some up if you don't have any favorite soup recipes already.

Happy Souping!

Chapter Two

Cleansing and Detoxifying Your Body

What is it? Why should I do it? How can I do it? What's in it for me? What are the benefits compared to other cleanses out there and are there any disadvantages of souping? In this chapter we will take a look and discover the answers to all these questions so you can weigh up the pros and cons for yourself.

What is Body Cleansing?

Body cleansing, also referred to, as detoxification is an age-old method of alternative medicine, dating back thousands of years. The premise of body cleansing is to rid your body of harmful toxins; chemicals and impurities that, if left to build up over time, can cause chronic pain, illness and a variety of life-altering ailments.

Detoxification History

While several forms of detoxification such, as reflexology, acupuncture, etc., have been used for centuries around the globe, a more recent form, emerging around the mid-1900s has become more prevalent. This more modern type of detoxification is more focused on cleansing the body through forms of diet alterations such as types of fasting and flushing away toxins through coercing and encouraging the bodies removal of waste. The main principal of fasting is avoiding solid foods and consuming only liquids of various types for certain periods of time. A balanced cleanse or fast is believed to flush toxins and impurities from our bodies and internal organs, giving them a chance to rest, therefore improving our overall health.

Why Do I Need to Cleanse?

There are numerous reasons why cleansing is presumed to be essential for our health and well being. It is inevitable that over time our bodies become overloaded with poisonous toxins and these toxins can cause disease, weight gain, circulatory issues, and overall life-altering health issues, but these ailments can be reduced and even eliminated entirely by regularly cleansing our bodies. One of the more common uses of body cleansing is weight loss, cleaning out our systems, boosting energy and basically kick-starting a more successful weight loss program.

Types of Cleansing

Body/Organ Cleanses Versus Liquid Cleanses

There are countless forms of body cleansing and detoxification with new and improved trends, fads, and miracle cures surfacing constantly. A few of the more tried-and-true forms that have been researched, tested, endorsed by medical professionals, recommended by celebrities, and having proven success rates include, but are not limited to the following:

Body/Organ Cleanses
- Colon Cleanse
- Kidney Cleanse
- Liver Cleanse
- Full-Body Cleanse

Liquid Cleanses

Liquid cleanses, one of the more popular types of cleansing, are based on the concept that no solid food is consumed during the designated time period, only the liquid of choice.

Water Detox

Water detox is the simplest form of liquid cleansing, consisting of only drinking water, although its success is based solely on drinking exact amounts of water at specific times, paying particular attention to avoiding over- or under-drinking. The purpose of this cleanse is to serve as a 'clean detox', giving you a clean, light feeling by flushing harmful toxins out of your system through the urinary tract. It is common to use this cleanse at the start of a weight loss program to eliminate excess water weight.

Juice Cleanse/Detox

Juice detox has become very popular as juicing machines or juicers have become more advanced and efficient. Fresh fruits and vegetables are simply put in the juicer, pureed together, and consumed. There is no heating, cooking, processing, chemicals, preservatives, etc.

Master Cleanse

The Master Cleanse also referred to, as the Lemonade Diet has been around longer than most of the liquid cleanses, dating back to 1940. The developer and author of the book, "The Master Cleanser" stated in his book "This diet will prove no one needs to live with their diseases. A lifetime of freedom from disease can become a reality." The premise of this cleanse is that the specifically prepared lemonade concoction includes enough calories and nutrients to not only cleanse an individual's digestive system, naturally encouraging healing, it has been proven suitable for weight loss and approved and endorsed by millions of people from around the world.

Milk Fasting

Milk fasting, as the name infers, is a type of cleanse in which only raw milk and water are consumed. This cleanse has not been tested to the extent of some other liquid cleanses, however, an article posted on the website 'Cooking God's Way' called "30 Day Raw Milk Fast" recounts the results of the experiment performed by Jeff, the man who decided to test the effectiveness of the cleanse. He had to drink up to a gallon of raw milk per day to even come close to the nutritional requirements for his body type. From the beginning and through the entirety of the cleanse, Jeff experienced high energy levels, lower blood pressure numbers, small amounts of weight loss, and didn't feel hungry. He did, however experience some bowel issues at the end of the second week due to a few necessary nutrients that the raw milk did not provide enough of, but with supplements the issues subsided. The only other adverse effect he experienced was a lack of energy on the first day after re-introducing solid food into his diet, but this was presumed to be due to the fact that his body had to become re-acclimated with using higher energy levels to digest solid food. Overall, Jeff felt like the fast was a success, giving him softer skin, a stronger mental outlook, and generally feeling 'well' throughout the entire month.

Beer Fasting

The beer fasting diet, while sounding rather comical or made-up, actually originated with the Monks, who vowed to only drink beer, a homemade brew, during the season of lent. The proposed purpose for this fast was to inspire increased awareness and spirituality among the Monks. This fast is not highly recommended by modern medical professionals, nor is it effective for weight less or increased awareness and spirituality.

Soup Detox or 'Souping'

Souping, or soup detox is a form of a liquid cleanse with the premise still being the consumption of only the one product, being soup. Experts claim that souping helps boost weight loss, increase energy, and even give your skin an added glow. The difference, and according to some professionals, the benefit to souping over juice detox is that instead of only containing raw fruits and vegetables, the soup additionally includes some processed ingredients, containing carbohydrates, fiber, and protein that the juices don't contain. There are a variety of soup recipes and types to choose from, including broth-based, cream-based, purees, and soups with grains and pastas. This variety and the added heartiness in some of the soups is believed to play a large role in the preference of the soup detox over the juice detox as the soups and the extra ingredients used makes individuals feel fuller longer and not have as many cravings for solid food.

Benefits and Disadvantages to Cleanses, Detoxes, and Fasts

As with any diet, procedure, alternative form of medicine, or any health-related topics, there are benefits and disadvantages to all the forms of cleansing, just as there are differing opinions of each by individuals experimenting and evaluating the results and the medical professionals who are developing and researching them.

Souping Versus Juice Detox

One of the big issues many people have with the modern soup detox is that it may simply be a trend: a fad that is popular for the moment but will not be a long-term accepted form of body cleansing. Alternatively, according to some researchers, souping is a healthier form of cleansing than juice detox due to one simple difference: soups retain fiber that is imperative to flushing impurities and toxins. In addition, the fiber content stabilizes blood sugar, making individuals feel less hungry. Another non-health related reason for souping preference is financial: it is cheaper to boil a big pot of broth, adding in a few vegetables and having a large amount to freeze and keep longer than it is to buy all the fresh fruits and vegetables needed to make one single glass of juice.

Juicing Advantages and Disadvantages

Consuming fresh, organic juices all day is beneficial to your digestive system as it allows it to rest as well as giving you the vitamins and nutrients your body needs. A disadvantage of only drinking juices with fresh fruits is the consumption of sugar. Some medical experts feel the sugar, without the fiber and protein to balance it out may be too high a level to be healthy. An alternative to juices made mostly from fruit, therefore higher in sugar content, is 'green juice'. Green juice is made of vegetables such as broccoli, kale, collards, or leafy greens, which means lower sugar and is a huge benefit to individuals who have problems getting the recommended servings of vegetables in a day. Most green juice provides up to 2 servings of fruits and vegetables per bottle so it is a healthy alternative to fruit-only juice. The downside is that by juicing the vegetables, the fiber is being 'stripped' due to being found in the pulp and skins, however you can physically add the pulp back in to the juicer or even add fiber & protein powders. Additionally, to add extra protein, you can crack a raw egg into your juicer and blend it in with the juice, actually thickens the drink and adds 3 to 5 times more nutrients than normal juices.

Medical Professionals Question Necessity of Cleansing/Detox

According to "Shape Magazine", a multiple-day, juice-only detox diet doesn't seem essential or even necessary for individuals as our bodies are designed to naturally rid themselves and detox through our organs including the liver, the GI tract, and the kidneys. Additionally, there is no scientific evidence to imply that our bodies truly need assistance in terms of ridding ourselves of waste, so it is generally not recommended to replace a normal, well-balanced food diet with a juice, soup, or liquid diet.

Chapter Three

Recipes

Are you looking for some healthy and tasty meals to promote detoxing as well as weight loss? There are so many recipes to try and start a brand new lifestyle. A decision to improve not only your health as well as to lose a few pounds it is best to start preparing your mind as well as your body.

The key to any lifestyle change is to make a commitment to yourself and once a commitment has been made, a reward. A reward system in place will keep you in line for what is most important to you and that is becoming a healthier you.

Healthy foods do not have to taste awful. What recipes shall be incorporated into a new fit you? There a large variety of recipes to try. For example, soups are your best friends. A great deal of them are broth based and are loaded with plenty of vegetables.

Creamy Vegan Cauliflower Soup W/ Kale Garlic Drizzle

Ingredients:

- 4 tbs. olive oil
- 1 cauliflower (cut out core, use just florets)
- 1 diced red onion

- 4 cloves raw garlic, peeled, slice thin
- 1/4 tsp garlic salt
- 1 32 oz can vegetable broth
- 1 cup kale leaves
- 1 lemon (juice & zest)

Method:

In a large stockpot over medium heat add ½ the olive oil. Once oil is heated, combine cauliflower, ½ the garlic and diced onions, and garlic salt. Stir ingredients over medium heat for 3-4 minutes. Once onions begin to brown and cauliflower is browned and beginning to soften, pour the broth slowly into the pan. Stirring occasionally, bring the contents to a simmer, still over medium heat. Cover the pot and keep cooking on medium till the cauliflower is soft (approx. 10 min.). Once the cauliflower is tender, blend small batches of contents, carefully, in a blender, OR, if using an immersion blender, cautiously blend entire contents. Blend until it is smooth.

Prepare Kale Drizzle:

In blender, combine kale leaves, olive oil (remaining ½), juice & zest from lemon, and the rest of the garlic. Blend on medium speed, processing until the mixture is smooth. Place soup in bowl, drizzle kale mixture over contents and serve immediately.

Creamy Tomato Soup with Basil

Ingredients:

For the soup

- 3 tbsp. butter
- 4 pounds tomatoes
- 4 medium onions
- 4 medium carrots
- 5 stalks celery
- 10 cloves garlic
- 4 cups Asian Vegetable broth
- 5 tbsp. tomato paste
- 10 tbsp. fresh basil
- 3 cups half and half
- 3 cup parmesan cheese
- 4 tsp. freshly ground black pepper
- 4 tsp. salt or to taste

For the Asian Vegetable Broth

- 2 medium onions (Chopped finely)
- 12 tbsp. fresh chives (Chopped)
- 4 carrots (Chopped)
- 4 celery ribs (Chopped)

Souping

- 6 cloves garlic (You will need to peel the garlic and cut the cloves finely)
- 2 sweet red peppers (Chopped finely)
- 6 tbsp. fresh ginger (You will need to peel and chop the ginger finely)
- 7 baby bok choy (These are also called Shanghai Tips. You will need to cut them into half)
- 4 stalks lemongrass (Remove the outer leaves and chop finely)
- 2 tsp. black pepper
- 2 tbsp. Kosher salt

Method:

For the Asian vegetable broth

You will need to wash all the vegetables well and prepare them. Now, place a stockpot on medium flame and add a little oil to the pot. Add the onions to the pot and sauté till they have turned golden brown and are translucent. Now, add the remaining ingredients to the pot and add the water making sure that all the vegetables are covered with the water. Add the seasoning to the pot and cover it.

Bring the stock in the pot to a boil. Now, reduce the flame and continue to simmer the ingredients in the pot. Do this after you have removed the cover from the pot. You will need to allow the broth to cool right before you drain the stock. You will need to use this broth in the soup.

For the soup

The first thing you will need to do is to core the tomatoes and peel all of them. Cut the tomatoes into quarters and set them aside. You will need to peel the onions and dice them finely.

You will also have to dice the carrots and the celery finely and also mince the garlic. Now, shred the Parmesan cheese and set all the ingredients aside.

You will need to place a saucepan on medium flame and wait for the pan to heat. Once it is hot, add the butter to the pan and once it has melted, you will need to add the onions to the pan. You will need to sauté the onions till they have turned golden brown and have become translucent and soft. You will also need to add the carrots and the celery to the pan.

Add the stock to the pot and the seasoning to the pot along with all the vegetables and cook all the ingredients well together. You will need to cover the pan and also cook the ingredients on high flame for at least thirty minutes. Once the time is up, you will have to uncover the pan and transfer the ingredients in the pan to a blender and blend till the soup has thickened and the texture is smooth. Ladle the soup into a bowl and garnish with the half and half and the Parmesan cheese and serve hot.

Beans and Greens Detox Soup

Broccoli and beans do not sound like a good combination together but however you will be amazed of how well they complement each other. Vitamins are essential to any meals. Vitamin K and C are great sources of providing nutrients to their body. This dinner has other benefits such as it is full of protein and is one of the many variations in detoxing soups out there on the market.

Ingredients:

- 1 large head of broccoli, chopped
- 5 cloves of garlic
- 1 to 1 1/2 cups spinach
- 1 1/2 lemons, juiced
- 1 large bunch of cilantro
- 1 can of cannellini or great northern beans, drained
- 2 tsp. turmeric
- 1 packet ALOHA Daily Good Greens
- Olive oil
- 3 1/2 cups of water
- 1 bouillon cube
- Salt and pepper

Method:

Before beginning any recipe, it is best to prepare your vegetables. The onions, and garlic need to be finely chopped and added to a stockpot that has olive oil. A dash of salt to the onions and garlic is all the seasoning you need at the moment. The stove needs to be on medium heat to cook the mixture till it reaches the aromatic stage, which usually will take no more than a minute or two. Broccoli that has been previously chopped is now ready to join the aromatic ingredients.

When spinach is added to the stockpot, do not worry about adding too much. The leaves will soon wilt. A can of drained beans with the following ingredients such as, turmeric powder, cilantro, bouillon, lemon and water will be the last fixings to join the crew. From time to time the mixture needs to be stirred to prevent it from sticking to the bottom of the large pot. Burnt soup will not taste good.

Within fifteen to twenty minutes of allowing all the ingredients to marry one another on low to medium heat, the soup will be ready for consumption. The stockpot should be removed the heat to prevent from the soup from being overcooked.

Souping

Susie Campbell

Diet Cabbage Soup

Ingredients:

- 1/2 Cabbage Head
- 1 Bunch of Celery
- 2 Onions
- 3 Carrots
- 2 Green Peppers
- 2 Tomatoes
- 1/4 Lemon
- Salt, Pepper and other spices

Method:

A pot of water needs to be brought boil so chopped celery; cabbage and tomatoes can be added. Each ingredient can be purchased from the local grocery store already prepared for you. This may cost more in the long run but however it will save you time in the kitchen.

While those are cooking in the boiling water, the next process can begin. A small frying needs to be heated up to a medium heat with a little bit of oil, so grated carrots and onions can stew together for a minutes. You can either cook the onions together with the carrots till they turn a bit yellow or do the onions first than the carrots. Either way is fine. Peppers will be the last ingredients to join the frying pan. These should cook for a few additional minutes.

When the frying pan fixings have reached their ultimate desire of taste and appearance, they will join the boiling water mixture. Each vegetable will cook till they reach their tender stage. Additional seasonings such as lemon juice, salt/pepper will be added to the pot. These will help to give the cabbage soup rich flavors. Sometimes cabbage can be too bland and needs a boost of flavoring.

Diet Beetroot Soup

Beets are not a favorite of many, especially me. However, it is good for you. This vegetable will not only leave your hands stained from their bright colored skins, but leaving you feel healthier.

Ingredients:

- 1 Large Beetroot
- 1 Large Carrot
- 1 Potato
- 1 Onion
- 1 Can of Peas
- Small can of tomato paste
- 1/4 Cabbage Head
- 1/2 Lemon
- 2 Bay Leaves
- Salt, Pepper and other spices

Method:

Bay leaves and chopped potatoes will be added to a boiling pot of water. A frying pan will fry the vegetables such as chopped onions with oil to prevent them from sticking to the base of the pan. The onions should be the color of yellow before adding the grated beetroot with carrot. Fifteen minutes of stewing time will allow the vegetables to reach a tenderization stage.

A separate bowl is required to add the tomato paste with two cups of hot water. This mixture will be added to the frying pan after it has been the fifteen minutes. All the ingredients should be stewed for an additional fifteen minutes.

Souping

Once these two tasks have been completed the frying pan ingredients can join the boiling pot mixture. A cabbage needs to be chopped and added along with peas. Lemon juice with one tbsp. of sugar is added at the end. Salt and pepper are seasonings to give the soup flavor. Additional spices can be added; it all depends on what you like. The soup should cook for about ten minutes.

Cottage Cheese and Kale Soup

Ingredients:

For the soup

- 4 packets cottage cheese
- 2 cups shredded Colby Jack cheese
- 3 tbsp. olive oil
- 3 medium onions (You will need to peel the onions and chop them finely)
- 6 cloves garlic (Peel the garlic well and mince it. you could crush the garlic if you do not like biting into garlic)
- 10 cups beef stock (This is to add the essence of protein to your dish)
- 2 bay leaves (You will need to remove this once you are done with the cooking)
- 1 15-ounce can diced tomatoes (If the tomatoes have been stored in their juice, you do not have to worry too much. if they have been preserved in a different way, you will need to drain the tomatoes and rinse them.)
- 1 15 ounce can chickpeas (You have to drain the chickpeas and rinse them well)
- 8 medium Yukon gold potatoes (You will need to peel the potatoes and cut them into cubes)
- 2 cups baby kale (You will need to tear the kale)
- Salt and pepper to taste

Souping

For the beef stock

- 2 pounds bones of beef
- 10 onions (peeled and halved)
- 10 carrots (Peeled and cut finely)
- 10 potatoes (Peeled and cut finely)
- 1 cup broccoli florets
- 2 cups cauliflower florets
- 8 Bay leaves
- 10 stalks celery
- 10 sprigs thyme
- 4 tsp. peppercorns
- Parsley stems
- 6 cloves garlic (You will need to peel the cloves and also chop them finely)

Method:

For the Beef Stock

The first thing you will need to do is to preheat the oven to 400 degrees Fahrenheit. While the oven is getting ready, you have to take the bones of the beef into a pan and cook them till the beef bones have turned brown. If there is any fat that is in the pan, you will need to leave the fat aside. This can be done in less than an hour. Make sure that you remove the bones of the pan the minute they have turned brown.

Add onions to the pan and cook them with the fat that is in the pan. You will need to sauté the onions till they have turned golden brown and are translucent. Add the other vegetables to the pan and cook them well too. Ensure that the vegetables have either turned brown or have become soft.

When this happens, you will need to remove the pan from the flame.

Take a stockpot and add water to it. Add the vegetables to the pot and make sure that the water covers the vegetables completely. Add the roasted bones of beef to the pot and place the stockpot on a medium flame. You will need to let the water in the pot boil. When the water has boiled, you will need to leave the pot on the flame to let the ingredients in the pot simmer. Add the herbs to the pot and continue to simmer. You will need to remove any fat that settles at the top of the stockpot during the cooking. When the stock thickens, you will have to add more water to it. Strain the stock and leave the stock aside for your soup.

For the soup

The first thing you will need to do is work on the cottage cheese. Clean the cheese well and remove any juice that may be on the cottage cheese. You will have to leave the cottage cheese aside. Now work on the onions and on the garlic. The other thing you could do with the garlic is to squeeze it to remove the flavor.

Place a pan on medium flame and add the oil to the pan. When the oil has warmed, you will have to add the onions and the garlic paste to the pan and sauté till the onions have turned golden brown and are translucent. Continue to stir the ingredients till the onions have become soft. Add the shredded cheese and the cottage cheese to the pan and continue to stir the ingredients. You will need to cook the ingredients till the cottage cheese cubes have turned brown on all sides and have a crisp outside. Make sure that you do not burn the cottage cheese or the shredded cheese. Add the vegetables to the pan and continue to cook them. You will need to add the beef stock to the pan when the vegetables have turned brown. Add the bay leaves to the pan and continue to cook the ingredients on high flame.

Cover the pan and continue to cook the ingredients for a minute or two. You will need to ensure that the ingredients in the pan have come to a boil. When the ingredients begin to boil, you will need to cover the pan and continue to simmer the ingredients. Uncover the lid of the pan and remove the bay leaves. When the soup has thickened, you will need to add the chickpeas and stir the ingredients well. Ladle the soup into bowls and serve it hot.

Diet Lentils Soup

Ingredients:

- 1 Cup of Lentils
- 6 1/4 Cups of Water
- 2 Tomatoes
- 2 Carrots
- 1 Onion
- 1/2 Lemon
- Salt, Pepper, Cumin and other spices

Method:

A pot of water needs to come to a boil. This will be start of the soup. Lentils will be an addition to the water. For the moment, chopped onions will be stewed in a frying pan that had been sprayed with a little bit of oil. Onions will turn a bit yellowish when cooked; this will be the perfect time for the grated carrots and chopped tomatoes to be added with the onions. The ingredients need to stew together and soak up each other's flavors.

The pot mixture and the frying pan mixture needs to come together in the stockpot. Grated carrots and chopped tomatoes will be the two final ingredients to the stockpot of fixings. When these two steps are combined, they need to be placed into a blender. This will create the soup into a puree.

Ginger and Butternut Squash Soup

Ingredients:

For the soup

- 10 lb. Butternut Squash
- 2 sprigs Sage
- 2 large Onions
- 4 two inches Fresh Ginger
- ½ tsp. Nutmeg
- Olive Oil
- 10 cups Vegetable Stock
- Salt and pepper to taste
- 1 ½ cups Squash seeds

For the Vegetable broth

- 12 cloves garlic
- 6 cups water
- 5 – 6 carrots
- 10 potatoes
- 8 onions
- 8 celery stalks
- 3 sprigs Thyme
- 3 sprigs Rosemary
- 3 sprigs Sage

- Fresh parsley
- Sea Salt
- Pepper

Method:

For the Vegetable Stock

You will first need to chop the vegetables finely and leave them aside. Take a large stockpot and add the water to the pot. Now, add the cut vegetables to the pot and ensure that the water has covered the vegetables well. There is a possibility that you will need to add a little more water to immerse the cut vegetables fully under water. Now, add the herbs and the seasoning to the pot and mix the ingredients well together.

Place the pot on high flame and bring the water to a boil. While the water is boiling, you will need to stir the ingredient together to ensure that you obtain all the nutrients required from the vegetables. When the water has boiled for five minutes, you will need to lower the flame and let the water continue to simmer. You will need to wait till the water has become slightly thick. Taste the stock to understand if the flavor is right for you. Strain the stock from the vegetables and set it aside for the soup.

For the soup

First peel the butternut and remove all the seeds from it. You will then need to cut the butternut into cubes of one inch each. Peel the onions and chop tem finely and leave them aside. Place a saucepan on a medium flame and add the oil to the pan when the pan is warm. When the oil is hot, add the onions to the pan and sauté till the onions have become golden brown and have become translucent.

Souping

Now you will need to add the sage, salt and the pepper to the pan. Mix all the ingredients together and remove the onions and keep them aside. Add the cubes of the butternut to the pan and cook the cubes till they have turned brown on all sides. This could take a minimum of ten minutes. Add all the other ingredients to the pan and cover it. Cook the ingredients on high flame for a few minutes.

Using an immersion blender, you will need to blend the ingredients in the pan into a smooth puree. You can add more of the stock if you want to change the consistency. Ladle the soup into serving bowls and serve hot.

Red Pepper and Edamame Soup

Baked red peppers and nutty edamame come together to build an appetizing aromatic meal.

Ingredients:

- 2 tbsps. Olive oil
- 1 cup of onion, cubed
- 3 tbsps. Garlic
- ½ cup roasted tomatoes, cubed
- 1 cup of baked red pepper, washed and dried
- 1/4 can chickpeas, washed and dried
- 3 cups of water
- 2 tbsp. parsley, cut
- 1/2 tsp salt

Method:

This soup involves a medium crockpot. Start by heating the oil over an intermediate heat for at least two minutes. Onions and garlic then to be cooked until the onions are see through.

Then take your tomatoes along with the baked red pepper, edamame and water and add them to the mixture. The heat needs to be greater than before and brought to a boil. Once it comes to a boil, the heat needs to be lowered and covered. It needs to simmer for ten minutes and then taken away from the heat.

The contents from the pot need to be placed in the blender and puree until it is completely smooth. Seasonings such as parsley salt, pepper blend them to incorporate them into the puree. It needs to be served hot.

Vietnamese Tofu Noodle Soup with Bok Choy

Ingredients:

For the Soup

- 4 cups Asian Vegetable Broth
- 1 packet rice noodles
- 2 cups tofu (You will need to chop the tofu finely or dice it, just the way you would like it)
- 2 cups Bok Choy
- Red pepper flakes
- Fresh Cilantro (chopped)
- 2 tsp. lemon juice
- 1 cup wild rice (Cooked)
- 1 cup Carrot (You will need to shred the carrots finely)
- 2 tbsp. peanuts (Chopped)
- 1 tbsp. soy sesame dressing
- 1 cup papaya

For the Asian Vegetable Broth

- 2 medium onions (Chopped finely)
- 12 tbsp. fresh chives (Chopped)
- 4 carrots (Chopped)
- 4 celery ribs (Chopped)
- 6 cloves garlic (You will need to peel the garlic and cut the cloves finely)

Souping

- 2 sweet red peppers (Chopped finely)
- 6 tbsp. fresh ginger (You will need to peel and chop the ginger finely)
- 7 baby bok choy (These are also called Shanghai Tips. You will need to cut them into half)
- 4 stalks lemongrass (Remove the outer leaves and chop finely)
- 2 tsp. black pepper
- 2 tbsp. Kosher salt

Method:

For the Asian vegetable broth

You will need to wash all the vegetables well and prepare them. Now, place a stockpot on medium flame and add a little oil to the pot. Add the onions to the pot and sauté till they have turned golden brown and are translucent. Now, add the remaining ingredients to the pot and add the water making sure that all the vegetables are covered with the water. Add the seasoning to the pot and cover it.

Bring the stock in the pot to a boil. Now, reduce the flame and continue to simmer the ingredients in the pot. Do this after you have removed the cover from the pot. You will need to allow the broth to cool right before you drain the stock. You will need to use this broth in the soup.

For the soup

Take a small pot and add the Asian vegetable broth to it and bring it to a boil. You will need to cook the noodles, the way it has been mentioned on the pack. In a small bowl, add the broth, noodles, tofu, and the bok choy that has been chopped. You will need to season the ingredients in the bowl with the cilantro, red pepper flakes and the lemon juice.

Susie Campbell

You will need to serve this with the wild rice and carrots. You will need to make this rice and carrot using the peanuts, carrot, wild rice and the soy sesame dressing. You will need to mix these ingredients well and serve them with the soup. You will need to serve the papaya as a dessert.

Mushroom Soup

This soup is rich in protein and has a velvety consistency. It is a robust amalgamation of mushrooms, Italian seasonings and freekah, which is a super grain.

Ingredients:

- 3 tbsps. of olive oil
- ½ cup of leeks, washed and dried
- ¼ cup of carrot, washed and dried and cut
- ¼ cup of celery, cut up
- 1 tbsp. garlic, cut up
- 1 tbsp. tomato purée
- ½ cup of shiitake mushroom
- ½ cup of chestnut mushroom
- 2 cups of water
- 2/3 cup of freekah, cooked
- 3 tbsps. Parsley, cut up
- ½ tbsp. of fresh rosemary, cut
- ¼ tbsp. of salt
- ¼ tbsp. of pepper
- ½ cup of cream

Method:

Traditional, easy and full of deliciousness. First, wash and prepare your mushrooms, ensuring that you get rid of all the hard parts, and then dice them up into small pieces. Take a saucepan and heat up a little oil. Place in it the celery, leeks, garlic, freekah, parsley, rosemary and mushrooms and then position a lid on top so that the ingredients can sweat for a few minutes. Take a tbsp. and take out four scoops of mushrooms and put to the side. Next, add the water and bring it to boiling point before lowering the heat and cook for

Susie Campbell

an addition 15 minutes. Add salt and pepper to your desired taste and then pour in the cream. Blend with your hand held blender and then bring back to the boil before pouring into a bowl. Top off with the mushrooms placed aside earlier.

Antique Grains Soup

Ingredients:

- 1 tbsp. of olive oil
- 1/3 cup of onion, diced
- ¼ cup of celery, diced
- ¼ cup of carrot, washed, dried and cut into slices
- 3 tsps of garlic
- 1 can diced tomatoes
- ¼ cup of amaranth, already cooked
- 1/3 cup of freekah, already cooked
- ¼ cup of quinoa, already cooked
- 1 ½ cups of water
- 2 tbsps. Parsley, cut
- ¼ tbsp. of salt
- ¼ tbsp. of pepper

Method:

You will need to warm up an ovenproof dish or pot for this recipe; the oil needs to be heated for two minutes before adding the onions, celery, carrots, and garlic for five minutes. Then add the tomatoes in the juice, amaranth, freekah, as well quinoa and the water. The heat needs to be increased and brought to a boil, which then needs to be lowered. Simmer it for fifteen minutes. Remove it from the heat and transfer to blender, add parsley and puree it smoothly.

Black Bean Soup

Ingredients:

- 16 tsp. Dried oregano leaves
- 4 tbsp. Salt (to taste)
- 8 cups dry black beans
- 6 tbsp. cumin
- 6 tbsp. oil
- 2 tsp. smoked paprika
- 20 cups Vegetable Broth
- 2 large bay leaves
- 2 onions
- 6 cloves garlic
- Cilantro (garnish)
- Sour Cream

Method:

You will first have to soak the beans in water or the vegetable stock and leave them out in the sun to dry. Now, chop the onions and the garlic coarsely and leave them aside. You will need to take a skillet and place it on medium flame. Add oil to the skillet and once the oil has warmed, add the onions and the garlic to the pan. You will need to sauté the onions till they have turned golden brown and are translucent and soft. You will need to continue to sauté when the garlic has turned golden brown too.

Now, add the powders to the pan along with the stock, bay leaves, oregano and the beans. Stir the ingredients well together and cover the skillet. Cover the skillet and increase the flame to high. Cook the ingredients for another ten minutes and uncover the skillet. Stir the ingredients in the skillet and continue to simmer till the liquid has thickened.

When the liquid has thickened, you will need to turn the heat off and remove the skillet from the gas. Set it aside and remove the bay leaves from the pan. You will need to mash the beans and transfer the ingredients to another bowl. Using an immersion blender puree the mixture till a smooth soup is obtained. Ladle the soup into bowls and garnish with cilantro and sour cream. Serve hot!

Susie Campbell

Red Lentil, Sweet Potato and Coconut Soup

Ingredients:

- 2 pounds of sweet potatoes
- 3 red onions
- ¾ tbsp. of cumin seeds
- ½ tbsp. of coriander
- Olive oil
- Four cloves of garlic, crushed
- One chili
- Fresh coriander
- ½ cup of red lentils
- 3 cups of vegetable stock
- One tin of light coconut milk
- One fresh lemon

Method:

The oven needs to be preheated to 180° degrees. The potatoes should be pared and cut into small chunks. Prepare and dice the onions into the same size wedges. Place veggies on a baking tray and sprinkle with cumin seeds, coriander seeds, pinch of sea salt and pepper for taste. Forty-five minutes will them lightly golden in color. Take a large saucepan over medium heat with oil poured in to fry the garlic, chili and coriander for two minutes till golden.

It is time to add the lentils, as well as the boiling stock and the coconut milk, which needs to be boiled. They need to cook for twenty minutes to cook them down. The veggies from oven can now be added to the mixture. Add the majority of the coriander and blended with hand held

Susie Campbell

blender till smooth. The rest of the leaves can now be added with toasted coconut slivers and squeeze of lemon juice.

Watercress soup

Ingredients:

- 2 potatoes
- 2 onions
- 2 cloves of garlic
- Olive oil
- ½ cup of organic stock
- 3 bunches of watercress

Method:

The potatoes, onions and garlic need to peeled and roughly chopped and tossed into a large frying pan that has been heated with a little bit of oil over medium heat. Stock needs to be added to the mixture when the onions have become translucent. Chopped watercress needs to be added once the potatoes have softened. Simmer for an additional three to four minutes. The soup can be liquefied with a hand held blender till it is silky smooth.

Susie Campbell

Tofu and Vegetable Soup

Ingredients:

For the soup

- 2 packets tofu (You will need to chop the tofu finely or dice them into cubes if that is how you like it better)
- 4 stalks celery (Chop the celery finely)
- 4 small onions (Chop the onions finely)
- 4 small carrots (Peel the carrots and chop them finely. You can grate the carrots if that is how you want to do it too.)
- 4 medium potatoes (Peel the potatoes and chop them into cubes of one inch each)
- 10 – 20 green beans (You will need to string the beans and also chop them into tiny pieces)
- 8 cups chicken stock (This will add the protein to the dish which will make you stronger)
- Salt and pepper to taste

For the chicken stock

- 2 pounds bones of chicken
- 10 onions (peeled and halved)
- 10 carrots (Peeled and cut finely)
- 8 Bay leaves
- 10 stalks celery
- 10 sprigs thyme
- 4 tsp. peppercorns

- Parsley stems
- 6 cloves garlic (You will need to peel the cloves and also chop them finely)

Method:

For the Chicken Stock

The first thing you will need to do is to preheat the oven to 400 degrees Fahrenheit. While the oven is getting ready, you have to take the bones of the chicken into a pan and cook them till the chicken bones have turned brown. If there is any fat that is in the pan, you will need to leave the fat aside. This can be done in less than an hour. Make sure that you remove the bones of the pan the minute they have turned brown.

Add onions to the pan and cook them with the fat that is in the pan. You will need to sauté the onions till they have turned golden brown and are translucent. Add the other vegetables to the pan and cook them well too. Ensure that the vegetables have either turned brown or have become soft. When this happens, you will need to remove the pan from the flame.

Take a stockpot and add water to it. Add the vegetables to the pot and make sure that the water covers the vegetables completely. Add the roasted bones of chicken to the pot and place the stockpot on a medium flame. You will need to let the water in the pot boil. When the water has boiled, you will need to leave the pot on the flame to let the ingredients in the pot simmer. Add the herbs to the pot and continue to simmer. You will need to remove any fat that settles at the top of the stockpot during the cooking. When the stock thickens, you will have to add more water to it. Strain the stock and leave the stock aside for your soup.

Susie Campbell

For the soup

Chop the onions, potatoes and the carrots very fine. Take a saucepan and add the oil to the pan. You will need to add the onions to the pan and cook them till they have turned golden brown and are translucent. Add the remaining vegetables to the pan and cook till they have all turned brown and are cooked through completely. Cover the pan and cook the ingredients on a very low flame. You will need to cook the ingredients this way for at least twenty minutes.

Add the tofu pieces to the pan and continue to cook the ingredients in the pan till the tofu has turned a little brown on all sides and has blended in well with the vegetables. Cover the pan one more time and cook the ingredients well. Add the stock to the pan and cook for another fifteen minutes. You will need to remove the tofu from the pan and place it on a plate. You will need to tear the tofu using a fork and transfer the tofu back into the pan. Continue to cook the ingredients in the pan for another fifteen minutes until the soup thickens. When the soup has thickened a little, ladle it into a bowl and serve the soup hot.

Pumpkin and ginger soup

Ingredients:

- 2 lbs. pumpkin
- 2 shallots
- 2/3 cup of ginger
- A few sprigs of fresh herbs, such as chives, mint
- Extra virgin olive oil
- Liter organic vegetable stock
- ½ cup of coconut milk, plus extra to serve
- ½ tbsp. chili powder
- 1 lime

Method:

The pumpkin will take some preparation, especially with deseeding it and giving it a rough chop. Shallots should be peeled and chopped. The ginger will be peeled and finely grated, which need to be sautéed in a frying pan with oil. The liquid ingredients such as the milk, coconut milk, and stock along with chili powder will be brought a boil for forty minutes. A food processor will be blitzing the ingredients to a smooth phase.

Spinach and Tortellini Soup

Ingredients:

- 4 1/4 Cups organic chicken or vegetable stock
- 2 fresh bay leaves
- ¾ cup of tortellini
- ¼ cup of frozen peas
- 1 large handful of spinach

Instructions:

Stock should be brought to a boil with bay leaves added to the stockpot. The tortellini will cook in the stock for four minutes till tender. The frozen peas can be added right to the stock; they will cook for at least three minutes. The spinach will be added last and will simply wilt as they cook. The soup can be served in large soup bowls.

Tofu and Vegetable Soup

Ingredients:

For the soup

- 3 packets tofu
- 10 – 12 cups frozen mixed vegetables
- 4 large onions
- 3 cans (14 ½ ounce each) stewed tomatoes (If the tomatoes have been stored in their juice, you do not have to worry too much. if they have been preserved in a different way, you will need to drain the tomatoes and rinse them.)
- 2 large russet potatoes
- 10 celery ribs
- 6 tbsp. canola oil
- 3 tsp. salt or to taste
- 3 tsp. pepper powder to taste
- 3 tsp. dried basil
- 10 cups pork stock, divided
- 4 cups instant rice
- 2 tbsp. Worcestershire sauce

For the pork stock

- 2 pounds bones of pork
- 10 onions (peeled and halved)
- 10 carrots (Peeled and cut finely)
- 10 potatoes (Peeled and cut finely)

- 1 cup broccoli florets
- 2 cups cauliflower florets
- 8 Bay leaves
- 10 stalks celery
- 10 sprigs thyme
- 4 tsp. peppercorns
- Parsley stems
- 6 cloves garlic (You will need to peel the cloves and also chop them finely)

Method:

For the pork Stock

The first thing you will need to do is to preheat the oven to 400 degrees Fahrenheit. While the oven is getting ready, you have to take the bones of the pork into a pan and cook them till the pork bones have turned brown. If there is any fat that is in the pan, you will need to leave the fat aside. This can be done in less than an hour. Make sure that you remove the bones of the pan the minute they have turned brown.

Add onions to the pan and cook them with the fat that is in the pan. You will need to sauté the onions till they have turned golden brown and are translucent. Add the other vegetables to the pan and cook them well too. Ensure that the vegetables have either turned brown or have become soft. When this happens, you will need to remove the pan from the flame.

Take a stockpot and add water to it. Add the vegetables to the pot and make sure that the water covers the vegetables completely. Add the roasted bones of pork to the pot and place the stockpot on a medium flame. You will need to let the water in the pot boil. When the water has boiled, you will need to leave the pot on the flame to let the ingredients in the pot simmer. Add the herbs to the pot and continue to simmer. You will need to remove any fat that settles at the top of the stockpot during the cooking. When the stock thickens, you will have to add more water to it. Strain the stock and leave the stock aside for your soup.

For the soup

The first thing you will need to do is to chop all the vegetables that have been given. You will need to peel the potatoes and then cut them into cubes of one inch each. The onions will need to be peeled and then cut finely. You will need to cut the tofu into small cubes of an inch. Place a saucepan on medium flame and add the oil to the pan when it has heated well. Once the oil is warm, you will need to add the tofu to the pan and make sure that the cubes have browned on all sides. Remove the tofu from the pan and leave it aside to cool.

Now, add the onions to the pan and sauté till the onions have turned golden brown and have become soft and translucent. Next, add the stock and the tomatoes to the pan and stir all the ingredients well together. Add the seasoning to the pan along with the sauce and stir the ingredients well. You will need to taste the soup to adjust the flavor.

Cover the pan and leave it on medium flame for at least twenty minutes. Once the timer has gone off, you will have to uncover the lid of the pan and add the frozen vegetables to the pan. You can let the ingredients in the pot simmer so that the soup thickens. When the soup has thickened, you will need to add the tofu cubes to the pan and ladle the soup into bowls and serve hot.

Susie Campbell

Summery Pea Soup with Turmeric Scallops

Ingredients:

For the pea soup

- 1 bunch of spring onions
- 1 clove of garlic
- 1 inch piece of ginger
- 1 fresh green Bird's-eye chili
- 1 tsp. cumin seeds
- Groundnut oil
- 3 fresh curry leaves
- 3 cups of organic vegetable or chicken stock
- 2 cups of fresh or frozen peas
- ½ tsp. jaggery or brown sugar
- 2 tsp. tamarind paste
- ½ a lime

For the turmeric scallops

- Groundnut oil
- ½ tsp. mustard seeds
- ¼ tsp. ground turmeric
- 10 fresh curry leaves
- ½ cup of queen or other small scallops

Method:

Spring onions are simple to trim and given a rough chop. The chili needs to be deseeded and chopped as well before being added. In a dry pan toast, the cumin seeds for a few short minutes. Add two tbsp. of oil, spring onions, garlic, ginger, and chili and curry leaves; fry for about two minutes. When it starts to sizzle, the stock should be poured into the stockpot.

Tortellini in brodo

Ingredients:

- 1 ½ cups of beef brisket
- 2/3 cup of beef shank bones
- 1 cup of free-range chicken thighs and drumsticks, skin on
- ½ an onion
- 1 stick of celery
- 1 carrot

For Pasta dough

- ¾ cup of flour, plus extra for dusting
- 2 large free-range eggs

For the Filling

- Olive oil
- 1/3 cup of prosciutto di Parma
- ¼ cup mortadella di Bologna
- 1 pinch of ground nutmeg
- ¼ cup of Parmesan cheese, plus extra to serve

Method:

A stock is made with the beef brisket bones, chicken, peeled onion and celery in a large stockpot. Carrots cut in half should be added to the pot. The next step is to submerge the vegetables with water and to cover the pot with a lid. Let it simmer for four hours, skimming it occasionally.

Prepare the pasta dough by blending the ingredients together either by hand or in a processor. Soft dough will form and should be wrapped in cling film for thirty minutes to rest. The mince shall be seasoned and fry in an oil till golden brown. Drain any excess oil from the meat.

The prosciutto, mortadella and nutmeg needs to be blitz in blender till its pulsed, and finely grated. Lightly dust a tray with flour

Timeless Minestrone

Ingredients:

- 4 rashers higher-welfare smoked streaky bacon
- 2 red onions
- 2 cloves of garlic
- 2 carrots
- 2 sticks of celery
- 1 bulb of fennel
- ½ a bunch of fresh basil
- Olive oil
- ½ cup of red wine
- 2 courgettes
- 1 cup of savoy cabbage or chard
- 2 x 400 g tins of chopped tomatoes
- 1 x 400 g tin of cannellini beans
- 3 cups of organic chicken or vegetable stock
- 1/3 cup of dried pasta (shells or odd ends)
- Extra virgin olive oil
- Parmesan cheese

Method:

The base of the soup is created by frying off the aromatic ingredients. Peel/chop the vegetables and stir into a pan of hot oil, gently sautéing them for at least twenty minutes is tender but yet hasn't changed appearance. Wine will flavor the veggies as it comes to a boil, now it's time to add the tomatoes and courgettes. Mix the cabbage, beans and juice with the stock. It needs to come to a boil. Pasta is added last to the pot. Allow it to cook. If it is too thick, add stock. Season to taste, drizzle basil leaves and Parmesan cheese for flavor.

Cream of Mushroom Soup

Ingredients:

For the soup

- 2 medium sized shallots (You will need to ensure that when you mince the shallots, you obtain two cups full)
- 5 tbsp. olive oil (You could choose to use butter, but it is best to use olive oil since it is healthier)
- 5 tbsp. whole wheat flour
- 6 cups Asian vegetable stock
- 2 pounds mushroom (You will need to chop the mushroom coarsely)
- 1 tbsp. seasoning salt
- 1 tbsp. umeboshi vinegar
- Black pepper
- Parsley sprigs (Use these for garnish)

For the Asian Vegetable Broth

- 2 medium onions (Chopped finely)
- 12 tbsp. fresh chives (Chopped)
- 4 carrots (Chopped)
- 4 celery ribs (Chopped)
- 6 cloves garlic (You will need to peel the garlic and cut the cloves finely)
- 2 sweet red peppers (Chopped finely)

Souping

- 6 tbsp. fresh ginger (You will need to peel and chop the ginger finely)
- 7 baby bok choy (These are also called Shanghai Tips. You will need to cut them into half)
- 4 stalks lemongrass (Remove the outer leaves and chop finely)
- 2 tsp. black pepper
- 2 tbsp. Kosher salt

Method:

For the Asian vegetable broth

You will need to wash all the vegetables well and prepare them. Now, place a stockpot on medium flame and add a little oil to the pot. Add the onions to the pot and sauté till they have turned golden brown and are translucent. Now, add the remaining ingredients to the pot and add the water making sure that all the vegetables are covered with the water. Add the seasoning to the pot and cover it.

Bring the stock in the pot to a boil. Now, reduce the flame and continue to simmer the ingredients in the pot. Do this after you have removed the cover from the pot. You will need to allow the broth to cool right before you drain the stock. You will need to use this broth in the soup.

For the soup

Take a large pot and add the olive oil to the pot. Place the pot on medium flame and when the oil is hot, add the shallots to the pot. You will need to sauté the shallots till they have turned golden brown and are soft and translucent. Add the flour to the pot and stir till the flour has toasted.

Add one cup of the stock one at a time and whisk the ingredients in the pot using a blender. You will need to bring

Susie Campbell

the mixture in the pot to a boil and add salt to it and then simmer. Add the mushrooms to the stockpot and simmer the ingredients in the pot for thirty minutes. You will need to puree the ingredients in a blender and adjust the seasonings. Garnish the soup with the parsley and serve hot.

Baked Potato Soup

Ingredients:

- 3 large baking potatoes or leftover baked potatoes
- ½ stick of butter
- 1 onion
- 1 Parmesan rind, whatever size you have in the fridge, optional
- 6 1/4 Cups organic chicken or vegetable stock
- Sour cream
- 1 small bunch of fresh chives

Directions:

Leftover baked potatoes save you at least three steps. Prepare all veggies by peeling, and cutting them. Use melted butter instead of oil. Cook the Parmesan and cut potatoes for five minutes. Add the stock and bring to a boil. Turn down the heat and allow it simmer for thirty minutes. After removing the rind from the stock, puree it till smooth with a stick blender. Garnish with your favorite toppings.

Cream of Broccoli Soup

Ingredients:

For the soup

- 12 cups fresh broccoli florets
- 8 cups Lamb Stock (This is to add the essence of protein to your dish)
- 8 cups milk
- 2 cups sour cream or low fat yogurt to serve
- 3 tsp. dried thyme
- Salt and pepper to taste

For the lamb stock

- 2 pounds bones of lamb
- 10 onions (peeled and halved)
- 10 carrots (Peeled and cut finely)
- 10 potatoes (Peeled and cut finely)
- 1 cup broccoli florets
- 2 cups cauliflower florets
- 8 Bay leaves
- 10 stalks celery
- 10 sprigs thyme
- 4 tsp. peppercorns
- Parsley stems
- 6 cloves garlic (You will need to peel the cloves and also chop them finely)

Method:

For the Lamb Stock

The first thing you will need to do is to preheat the oven to 400 degrees Fahrenheit. While the oven is getting ready, you have to take the bones of the lamb into a pan and cook them till the lamb bones have turned brown. If there is any fat that is in the pan, you will need to leave the fat aside. This can be done in less than an hour. Make sure that you remove the bones of the pan the minute they have turned brown.

Add onions to the pan and cook them with the fat that is in the pan. You will need to sauté the onions till they have turned golden brown and are translucent. Add the other vegetables to the pan and cook them well too. Ensure that the vegetables have either turned brown or have become soft. When this happens, you will need to remove the pan from the flame.

Take a stockpot and add water to it. Add the vegetables to the pot and make sure that the water covers the vegetables completely. Add the roasted bones of lamb to the pot and place the stockpot on a medium flame. You will need to let the water in the pot boil. When the water has boiled, you will need to leave the pot on the flame to let the ingredients in the pot simmer. Add the herbs to the pot and continue to simmer. You will need to remove any fat that settles at the top of the stockpot during the cooking. When the stock thickens, you will have to add more water to it. Strain the stock and leave the stock aside for your soup.

For the soup

You will first need to place a pan on medium flame and add every ingredient in the list to the pan except for the sour cream and the milk. You will need to mix the ingredients together and cover the pan and leave it on the medium flame. Do this for at least fifteen minutes.

Once the time is up, you will have to uncover the lid and leave the ingredients to cool. You have to use the immersion blender and blend all the ingredients together and add the milk to the pan and warm the soup once more. Once the soup has thickened, you have to ladle the soup into bowls and serve it hot garnished with a scoop of the sour cream.

Caprese Soup

Ingredients:

- 1 bulb of garlic
- 2 lb. mixed tomatoes
- Extra virgin olive oil
- 4 sun-dried tomatoes in oil
- 1 tbsp. soft brown sugar
- ¼ cup of basil leaves, plus a few extra to garnish
- 1½ tbsp. red wine vinegar
- 4 slices of sourdough bread
- 1 cup of buffalo mozzarella

Method:

Preheat the oven to two hundred degrees, while preparing the veggies by peeling and cutting. Roast them for twenty-five minutes with tomatoes and drizzle of oil on a tray. Squeeze the garlic out from its peel and into a blender with roasted tomatoes, dry tomatoes and seasonings till a smooth puree. Sourdough can be heated and charred to use as a dunking device when the soup is served at room temperature with a slice of mozzarella.

Susie Campbell

Caldo Verde

Ingredients:

- 1 large onion
- 2 cloves of garlic
- 2 pounds of potatoes
- 1 cup of kale or cavolo nero
- Extra virgin olive oil
- Paprika

Method:

Each vegetable should be cleaned, peeled and chopped for the preparation of the soup. Onions and garlic should be fried over medium heat till they are softened. After the liter of water is added, the potatoes can be as well. They will cook for about five minutes till they are softened too.

Seasoning the chorizo slices with paprika, fry them with a little bit of oil in a frying pan. Once they are cooked, they can be added to the soup. Ladle the soup into individual bowls and garnish them with bit of oil and a side of corn bread.

Celeriac Soup

Ingredients:

For the soup

- 4 tbsp. olive oil
- 2 pounds onions (You will need to slice the onions finely)
- 2 tsp. salt
- ½ cup rolled oats
- 3 pounds celeriac (You will need to trim it and cut the celeriac into slices in the shape of a half moon. Make sure that these slices are half an inch in thickness)
- 6 cloves garlic (You will need to peel the garlic and chop the cloves finely)
- 10 cups vegetable stock
- 1 lemon (Zest the lemon and juice it out)
- Salt and Pepper to taste

For the Vegetable stock

- 12 cloves garlic
- 6 cups water
- 5 – 6 carrots
- 10 potatoes
- 8 onions
- 8 celery stalks
- 3 sprigs Thyme
- 3 sprigs Rosemary

- 3 sprigs Sage
- Fresh parsley
- Sea Salt
- Pepper

Method:

For the Vegetable Stock

You will first need to chop the vegetables finely and leave them aside. Take a large stockpot and add the water to the pot. Now, add the cut vegetables to the pot and ensure that the water has covered the vegetables well. There is a possibility that you will need to add a little more water to immerse the cut vegetables fully under water. Now, add the herbs and the seasoning to the pot and mix the ingredients well together.

Place the pot on high flame and bring the water to a boil. While the water is boiling, you will need to stir the ingredient together to ensure that you obtain all the nutrients required from the vegetables. When the water has boiled for five minutes, you will need to lower the flame and let the water continue to simmer. You will need to wait till the water has become slightly thick. Taste the stock to understand if the flavor is right for you. Strain the stock from the vegetables and set it aside for the soup.

For the soup

You will need to take a large stockpot and place it on medium flame. Add the onions to the pot along with the garlic. You will need to sauté the onions well till they turn golden brown and translucent. You will need to add the salt and the oats to the pot along with the celeriac. You will need to cover the pot and continue to cook the ingredients for ten minutes while you stir occasionally.

Add the stock to the pot and bring the ingredients in the pot to a simmer. Cover the pot and cook the ingredients for another thirty minutes. You will need to check on the celeriac and make sure that it is very tender. Transfer the ingredients to the blender and puree the soup till you obtain a smooth mixture. You will need to season the soup well with the salt, pepper and the lime juice and taste. Serve hot.

Hot Parsnip and Lentil Soup with Truffle Oil

Ingredients:

- 1 small smoked good quality ham hock
- 1 onion
- 3cm piece of ginger
- 3 cups of parsnips
- Olive oil
- 1 cup of red lentils
- 4 cups of organic vegetable stock
- A few sprigs of fresh mint
- Fat-free Greek yoghurt
- Truffle Oil

Method:

Place the ham hock into pot and submerge it with fresh cold water and then bring it to the boil before lowering the temperature. Allow the contents to simmer for 90 minutes or so before draining it. Put the ham hock to one side. Take the truffle oil and put it in a saucepan along with the olive oil, ginger and garlic; heat for about five minutes. Cut pieces of the ham up and place in the drained liquid. You can strain the oil if you wish before drizzling over the soup along with a bit of the fat free yoghurt and fresh mint.

Broccoli Soup

Ingredients:

- 1 clove of garlic
- 2 sticks of celery
- 1 ½ cups of broccoli
- Fresh mint
- Olive oil
- 3 cups of chicken or vegetable stock
- Ricotta cheese

Directions:

The garlic should be peeled and chopped finely. Celery and broccoli will be trimmed and chopped roughly. Oil heated in a pan will soften the garlic and celery, which will only take two or three minutes. Broccoli and stock should be added next. Cooking for five minutes, while a handful of mint leaves is being blitz in blender. Sprinkle garnish on top with a dollop of ricotta cheese.

Super Noodle Ramen with Kale and BBQ Mushrooms

Ingredients:

- One clove of garlic
- 1 large onion
- Olive oil
- Kale
- Two tbsp. of dark miso paste
- Two tbsp. of white miso paste
- One tbsp. of tahini
- One tbsp. of low-salt soy sauce
- Two tbsp. of mirin
- One tbsp. of sugar
- One tbsp. of white wine vinegar
- One chili
- 1 ½ cups of mixed mushrooms
- Four tbsp. of teriyaki sauce
- 1 cup of ramen noodles
- Four tbsp. of sesame seeds

Directions:

The broth is simple to make. The garlic cloves need to be peeled and roughly slice the onions. A splash of oil in a large skillet over a medium heat needs to cook the whole garlic and onion for at least thirty minutes. The lid needs to stay on the pan for another twenty minutes to keep the moisture from leaking out. On the final ten minutes, the lid can be removed to give the ingredients a little bit of color.

The liter of water should be added to the pan at this time. When the water comes to a boil, the heat needs to be reduced and brought to a simmer for twenty minutes. The oven needs to be preheated to 120° degrees.

The kale needs to be cleaned and prepared by removing any tough bits from the leaves. The proper way to toast the leaves is to place a portion of the leaves on a greased baking sheet for thirty minutes. This will ensure they are crispy and not over cooked. The kale leaves can be seasoned with salt and pepper for taste. They can be tossed with oil and spread out to make sure they do not overlap.

The broth needs to be strained through a cloth. The garlic and onion should be pressed with a large spoon to release the flavors back into the dish. Both miso pastes and the tahini need to be mixed in a small bowl. A little bit of broth will help loosen it up. This mixture will need to go back into the main pan and seasoned with soy sauce and mirin. The broth requires to be warm until everything else is ready.

The remaining kale will be blanched in the broth for about two minutes. The other batch will be pickled. When it is cool to the touch, it needs to be squeezed to release all the juice into the broth and place the kale in the bowl.

Mushrooms need to be sliced thickly and deep fried for about ten minutes. Teriyaki and a splash of oil is to keep them from moving too much in the pan till six or eight minutes are up. The noodles can be cooked in the broth, depending on the manufacturer's instructions. The moment everything is ready, the noodles and broth can be divided into four different bowls. The vegetables will be used for the garnishing. Toasted seeds will be sprinkled on top with a drizzle of sesame oil.

Pasta e Fagioli Soup

Ingredients:

- 6 tbsp. extra virgin olive oil
- 2 medium sized onions (Dice the onions fine. The cut onions should come to up to two cups)
- 2 medium sized carrots (You will need to dice them finely and ensure that he diced carrots fit about two cups)
- 5 stalks celery (You will need to dice them finely and ensure that he diced carrots fit about two cups)
- 6 medium sized garlic cloves (You will need to mince the garlic to ensure that it comes to up to two or three tablespoons)
- 2 28 ounce cans of plum tomatoes (You will need to puree the tomatoes to make sure that it comes to up to four cups)
- 6 cups vegetable stock (You can make the stock at home using the recipe mentioned above)
- One can of cannellini beans
- 4 bay leaves
- 2 tsp. fresh thyme (Mince it well)
- 1 tsp. sea salt
- ½ tsp. black pepper
- 3 cups whole wheat pasta

Method:

Souping

Take a large pot and add the oil to the pot. Place the pot over medium flame and add sauté till the onions have turned golden brown and translucent. Make sure that the onions are soft. Now, add the garlic to the pot and cook till the garlic has turned golden brown and gives a wonderful fragrance. You will need to cook this for five minutes.

Now, add the tomato puree to the pot along with the stock and the beans and bring the ingredients in the pot to a simmer. You will need to add the thyme, black pepper, salt and the bay leaves to the stock while you stir to ensure that the flavor has blended well. When you have simmered it, you will need to add the pasta to the pot and stir continuously till the pasta has been cooked evenly. You will need to do this for ten minutes and then remove the bay leaves. Garnish with grated cheese and serve hot.

Easy and Delicious Miso Soup

Ingredients:

- 2/3 cups of rice (can be brown, white or wild Rice)
- 1/8 cup of dried porcini mushrooms
- One onion
- Sesame oil
- A small piece of ginger
- ½ tbsp. of miso paste
- 2 ½ cups of chicken stock
- Six stalks of radishes
- Wine vinegar
- One cup of chicken breast, skinned and chopped
- Kale
- One sheet of nori
- 2/3 cup of various mushrooms

Method:

Start by washing your rice and straining the water away (this gets rid of all the unwanted starch – it will be white in color); repeat several times. Then place your rice in a saucepan and add water. Simmer until cooked. Then take your porcini into a bowl and add hot water so that your mushrooms become rehydrated.

Next, take your onion, peel and then chop into small pieces and then put them in a saucepan. Add a little sesame oil and brown the onions until they become gold. Then take the ginger; once it has been peeled then cut it into very small pieces. Lower the temperature and place the ginger, stock and miso into the saucepan before adding in the porcini (with the water it was placed in, but not the grainy part). Top the saucepan with its lid and allow to gently cook for 20 minutes. As this is cooking, take the radishes, cut them in half, and put in a bowl. Dash them with the vinegar and a sprinkling of salt.

Take the chicken and cut it into small pieces before cutting the kale and nori. Then cut some of the mushrooms into small pieces, but you can leave the nice ones whole, and pour them all into the soup. Then place the lid back over the saucepan for five minutes or until the chicken is cooked properly. Place some of the rice into bowls, along with the radishes, before pouring some of the soup into the bowls. Add salt and pepper to taste.

Turkey and Coconut Milk Soup

Ingredients:

- Two stalks of lemongrass
- Three shallots
- Two chilies
- One small piece of ginger
- Three coriander roots
- Two cups of turkey tock
- One tin of light coconut milk
- One tbsp. of soft brown sugar
- Three lime leaves
- ½ cup of oyster mushrooms
- 1 cup of cooked turkey with the skins taken off
- Two tbsp. Of fish sauce
- Half a lime
- Fresh coriander

Method:

Take the lemongrass and cut it appropriately before preparing the chilies and the shallots. Peel the ginger and then cut it into small pieces. Be sure to wash the coriander roots thoroughly if you intend to use them.

Pour the coconut milk and the turkey stock into a saucepan over a high temperature, bringing to the boil before lowering the heat. After this, combine the lemongrass, chilies, ginger, coriander roots, shallots and sugar with the contents in the saucepan. Add salt and pepper to taste and then place a lid on top and allow to cook on a low heat for four to six minutes.

Souping

Cut the turkey and the mushrooms into pieces and then place into the saucepan. Cook for an addition few minutes before placing the fish sauce and fresh lime juice. Pour into bowls and sprinkle some coriander leaves on the surface of the soup.

Susie Campbell

Cold Cucumber Soup

Ingredients:

- ½ stick of unsalted butter
- One onion
- Three fresh cucumbers
- Four cups of chicken stock
- Fresh chives
- Fresh parsley
- The juice of two lemons
- 1 cup of single cream

Method:

After peeling the onion and cutting it into small pieces, then wash and cut up your cucumbers. Then, start melting the butter in a saucepan and gently cook the onions over a low heat for around six minutes. After this, add the cucumbers and then lower the temperature. Cook the ingredients for another six minutes before pouring in the stock. Increase the temperature until it comes to boiling point and then quickly lower the temperature once more. Add salt and pepper to taste and continue to cook for another five minutes. The cut your chives and parsley and sprinkle into the saucepan, along with the juice of two lemons and cook for an additional five minutes. Then pour into a blender and puree until it becomes a silky consistency. You can either cool the soup by leaving out or you can place in the fridge to chill. Prior to serving, add the cream and stir in thoroughly.

Susie Campbell

Traditional Goulash Soup

Ingredients:

- 1 cup of diced onions
- Two bulbs of garlic
- One green pepper
- Two chopped tomatoes
- Fresh marjoram
- Olive oil
- 3 cups of chopped beef
- One tbsp. of paprika
- Four cups of beef stock
- 1 tbsp. of caraway seeds
- Red wine vinegar
- One tbsp. of tomato purée
- 1 pound of potatoes

Method:

Start by peeling the onions and then cut them into pieces before peeling the garlic and dicing them up. Wash and cut the pepper, removing all the seeds, before chopping the tomatoes and cutting the marjoram. Pour the oil into a saucepan over a medium heat and cook the onions, peppers and garlic before adding the beef. Cook everything until the meat is thoroughly cooked and then add the paprika. Carry on cooking for a few more minutes and then add ½ cup of the beef stock and allow it to come to boiling point and stay there until the mixture has been reduced. Then put in the caraway seeds, the tomato puree, the vinegar, tomatoes and marjoram into the saucepan along with the rest of the stock. Cover with a lid and leave for up to two hours. Then cut up your peeled potatoes and put them in the mixture and carry on cooking until the potatoes are done.

Creamy Tomato Basil Soup

Ingredients:

- 4 medium carrots (You will need to peel the carrots and dice them finely)
- 4 stalks celery (You will need to dice the stalks finely)
- 6 cloves garlic (You will need to peel the cloves and mince the cloves)
- 5 tbsp. butter
- 2 cups parmesan cheese (Shred the cheese finely)
- 3 cans (14.5 ounce) chicken stock
- 3 medium onions (You will need to peel the onions and dice them finely)
- 2 tbsp. fresh basil
- 3 cups half and half
- 2 tsp. freshly ground black pepper
- 4 pounds tomatoes (You will need to core the tomatoes, peel and cut them into halves or quarters)
- 2 tbsp. tomato paste
- 2 tsp. salt or to taste

Method:

You will need to take a saucepan and place it on medium or high flame. Now, add the butter to the pan when it is warm. Once the butter has melted, you will have to add the onions and the garlic to the pan. Sauté the onions and garlic till the onions have turned golden brown, translucent and soft and the garlic has turned golden brown. Next, add the carrots and the celery to the pan and stir-fry them.

Add the stock to the pan along with the tomatoes and the seasoning. You will have to ensure that you mix the ingredients well together. Cover the pan and turn the heat up. Cook the ingredients for fifteen minutes and then uncover the pan. When the liquid has thickened, you will need to remove the bay leaves. Using an immersion blender, you will need to obtain a mixture that is smooth. You will need to ladle the soup into bowls, garnish with the Parmesan and half and half and serve hot!

Creamy Carrot Soup with Oats

Ingredients:

For the soup

- 4 tbsp. extra virgin olive oil
- 2 large onions (You will need to dice them finely)
- 1 tsp. sea salt
- 4 pounds carrots (You will need to peel the carrots and cut them into circles that are half an inch each)
- 10 cups vegetable stock
- ½ cup oats (You could get the brand that you like most)
- 2 tsp. Lemon juice
- 3 tsp. ginger juice
- 4 tbsp. dill (This will need to be cut very finely since you will be using the dill for garnish)

For the Vegetable stock

- 12 cloves garlic
- 6 cups water
- 5 – 6 carrots
- 10 potatoes
- 8 onions
- 8 celery stalks
- 3 sprigs Thyme
- 3 sprigs Rosemary

- 3 sprigs Sage
- Fresh parsley
- Sea Salt
- Pepper

Method:

For the Vegetable Stock

You will first need to chop the vegetables finely and leave them aside. Take a large stockpot and add the water to the pot. Now, add the cut vegetables to the pot and ensure that the water has covered the vegetables well. There is a possibility that you will need to add a little more water to immerse the cut vegetables fully under water. Now, add the herbs and the seasoning to the pot and mix the ingredients well together.

Place the pot on high flame and bring the water to a boil. While the water is boiling, you will need to stir the ingredient together to ensure that you obtain all the nutrients required from the vegetables. When the water has boiled for five minutes, you will need to lower the flame and let the water continue to simmer. You will need to wait till the water has become slightly thick. Taste the stock to understand if the flavor is right for you. Strain the stock from the vegetables and set it aside for the soup.

For the soup

Take a medium sized pot and add a little oil to the pot. Place the pot over medium heat and wait till the oil has warmed up. When the oil warms, add the salt and the onions to the pot and sauté till the onions have turned golden brown and are translucent and soft. Make sure that they do not burn. Now, add the carrots to the pot and cover the pot while cooking the ingredients in the pot for five or ten minutes. You will need to stir the ingredients constantly to ensure that the vegetables do not turn brown.

Now, add the stock to the pot followed by the oats. You will need to increase the flame and bring the ingredients in the stock to a boil. When the stock has begun to boil, you will need to reduce the heat and let the ingredients continue to simmer. You will need to cover the pot and let the vegetables cook further, till the carrots have become very soft and tender.

Transfer the soup to a blender and blend till you obtain a mixture that is creamy. You can add a little more stock to the pot if you desire. Add the ginger and lemon juices to the soup and adjust the seasoning. Garnish with the chopped dill and serve hot!

Creamy Cauliflower soup with Kale Drizzle

Ingredients:

- 8 tbsp. olive oil
- 2 heads of cauliflower (You will need to cut them into florets)
- 2 red onions (Chopped finely)
- 6 cloves garlic (Peel the cloves cut them finely. Divide the cut garlic into two halves)
- ½ tsp. garlic salt
- 1 ½ 32 ounce cans vegetable broth (You could also make the broth using the recipe that has been given above)
- 2 cup Kale leaves
- 2 lemons (You will need to zest them and juice them)

Method:

Take a large stockpot and place it on a medium flame. When the pot has heated, you will need to add the olive oil to the pot and wait till it warms. When the oil is warm enough, you will need to add the onions and half the portion of the garlic to the pot and sauté till the garlic and the onions have turned golden brown. Make sure that the onions are very soft. Now, add the cauliflower florets to the pot and cook them till they have started to turn brown.

Next, add the broth to the pot and place it over medium flame and continue to simmer the broth. You will need to cover the pot and cook the ingredients till the cauliflower has become very tender. Transfer the ingredients from the pot into a blender and blend till you have obtained a very smooth mixture. You will now have to make the kale drizzle.

Add the olive oil, the lemon zest, lemon juice, kale leaves and the remaining garlic to the blender and process the ingredients till the mixture obtained is smooth. Add this drizzle over the soup and serve it immediately.

Souping

Miso Soup

Ingredients:

- 4 tbsp. sesame oil
- 2 medium sized onions (Try to ensure that they are not more than ten ounces)
- 2 carrots (Cut them into the shape of a matchstick)
- 4 ribs celery (Sliced diagonally)
- 10 shitake mushrooms (You will need to slice the mushrooms finely)
- 10 cloves garlic (You will need to peel the garlic and slice the garlic thin)
- 2 pieces kombu
- 2 tsp. salt
- ½ cup wakame (You will need to soak the wakame for ten minutes and then drain it)
- ½ cup arame (You will need to soak the wakame for ten minutes and then drain it)
- 1 lb. tofu (Make sure that you dice it well)
- 10 cups water
- 2 tbsp. ginger juice (You can take more of the juice if you want to too)
- 2 tbsp. lemon juice
- 2 tbsp. brown rice vinegar
- 2 cups white mellow miso (You could use more for taste)

- 4 scallions (Separate the white and the green parts of the scallion and chop them finely. You will need to use them for the garnishing)

Method:

Take a pot and add the oil to the pot. Now, add the onions to the pot along with the garlic and sauté. You will need to do this till the onions have turned golden brown and are translucent and soft. Add the celery, Kombu, salt, carrots and the shitake mushrooms to the pot and continue to sauté. You will need to cover the pot and cook the ingredients on low flame.

Now, add the wakame, tofu and the arame to the pot and continue to sauté the ingredients for another twenty minutes. Add the water to the pot and bring the water to a boil. You will need to lower the flame and uncover the pot and cook the ingredients for another fifteen minutes. Turn the heat off and leave the ingredients in the pot for some time. Add the lemon juice and the ginger to the broth and taste the broth. You will need to temper the miso in a bowl by adding to cups of the broth to one cup of the miso. When you have tempered the miso, add it to the soup pot. Garnish the soup with the scallions and serve hot.

Susie Campbell

Souping

White Bean Soup

Ingredients:

- 6 tbsp. olive oil (You will need to divide the oil into two halves)
- 2 lb. tofu or cottage cheese (Make sure that you have fresh tofu and cut either of the two into cubes or slices depending on how you like it)
- 4 large carrots (Chop them finely)
- 2 large onions (You will need to peel and chop the onions finely)
- 4 bay leaves (You will need to remove these the minute you finish cooking)
- 2 sprigs Fresh rosemary
- 3 cans cannellini beans (You will need to drain the beans and rinse them well if you are using beans from a can)
- 4 cloves garlic (You will need to peel the garlic and slice the garlic finely)
- 2 bunches of kale (You will need to chop the kale finely)
- 6 cups vegetable stock
- 2 cups shredded cheese

Method:

Take a large pot and place it on medium flame. You will need to add the oil to the pot and warm it. When the oil has warmed, add the tofu or cottage cheese cubes and stir them occasionally to ensure that they have browned on all sides.

This will take ten minutes or so. Add the vegetables and the bay leaves to the pot and continue to cook. You will then need to add the rosemary to the pot and continue to cook the ingredients pot till the onions turn golden brown and are translucent.

Now, add the beans and the garlic to the pot and cook all the ingredients together for at least ten minutes. Next, add the stock and the kale to the pot and season the ingredients in the pot with the black pepper and the salt. Cover the pot and bring the ingredients in the pot to a boil and reduce the heat and simmer the ingredients. This may take a minimum of half an hour. While the soup is simmering, you will need to get some bread ready to eat with the soup.

Broil the bread in a baking pan that has been greased with olive oil and salt. Once the broil has melted, you will need to top it with cheese and serve the bread along with the soup.

Souping

Spicy Chicken Tortilla Soup

Ingredients:

- 2 large onions (You will need to peel the onions and dice them finely)
- 4 tsp. coconut oil
- 2 large red peppers (You will need to dice them finely)
- 2 cups jalapenos (It is better if these are pickled jalapenos. You will need to cut them finely)
- 6 cloves garlic (Peel the garlic and mince the cloves well)
- 4 tsp. dried oregano
- 4 tsp. coriander (You will need to try and get some dried coriander)
- 4 tsp. ground cumin
- 4 tbsp. olive oil or ghee
- 6 cups tofu (You will need to cut the tofu finely or dice them if that is what you need)
- 6 cups Kale leaves (You will need to tear them well)
- 1000 grams canned tomatoes (You will need to drain and rinse the tomatoes well)
- 6 cups vegetable stock
- 4 lemons (You will need to zest these lemons and also juice the lemons)
- Salt and Pepper to taste
- 10 tbsp. pumpkin seeds (These will need to be roasted well)

- 4 large sized spring onions (When you chop the onions, you will need to make sure that it fills at least three cups)
- 10 tbsp. Fresh cilantro leaves
- 3 avocados (You will need to slice the avocado finely)
- 1 tsp. paprika

Method:

You will need to take a large saucepan and place the pan on a medium flame. You will need to add the oil to the pan and when it is warm, you will need to add the onions to the pan and sauté till the onions have turned translucent and are golden brown. When the onions have become soft, you will need to add the red peppers to the pan and cook till the peppers have become soft too.

Once the onions and the red peppers are soft, add the garlic, jalapenos, oregano, the cumin and the coriander powders to the pan and cook till you have a lovely fragrance filling your kitchen. You will now have to add the stock, lime juice, tomatoes, tofu, lime zest and the salt to the pan and taste the flavor. You will need to increase the heat and bring the ingredients in the pan to a boil. Cover the pan and let the ingredients simmer. Once the soup has thickened, you will need to ladle the soup into a bowl and serve garnished with cilantro, avocado and the green onions. Sprinkle the pumpkin seeds over the garnish and serve it warm.

Pizza Soup

Ingredients:

- 3 packets tofu
- 10 ounces slices of cottage cheese (You will need to slice them into halves)
- 3 tbsp. olive oil or ghee
- 2 large onions (You will need to peel the onions and dice them finely. Now, separate the diced onions into two halves)
- 2 red bell peppers (Chop them finely)
- 12 mushrooms (Make sure that you chop them finely)
- 4 cloves garlic (You will need to peel the garlic and chop the garlic finely)
- 10 sprigs thyme
- 3 cans tomatoes (If the tomatoes have not been stored in their own juices, you will need to rinse the tomatoes well with water after you drain the tomatoes)
- 3 cans tomato paste
- 4 cans vegetable stock
- 3 cans black olives
- 2 cups water
- Red pepper flakes (You can add these to add taste)
- Salt and pepper to taste

Method:

Place a large saucepan or a large pot on a medium flame and place it over a medium flame. You will need to add the olive oil or ghee to the pan and when the ghee melts or the oil warms; you will need to add the garlic, thyme and half of the chopped onions. You will need to sauté till the onions have turned golden brown and translucent. You will now need to add the tomatoes, the tomato paste and the water to the pan and bring the ingredients to a boil.

Reduce the heat and simmer the ingredients in the pan for thirty minutes. You will need to remove the pan from the heat and transfer the ingredients into a blender. Blend the ingredients to obtain a smooth mixture that will then again have to be transferred into the saucepan.

Take a saucepan and add the olive oil to the pan. When the oil has warmed, you will need to add the tofu and the cottage cheese to the pan and cook till the tofu and cottage cheese slices have browned on all sides. Now, add the remaining onions to the pan and sauté till they have turned golden brown and translucent. Now, add the mushrooms to the saucepan and sauté. Transfer all these ingredients to the first saucepan and place the pan on medium heat. You will need to simmer the ingredients and wait till the soup thickens. Ladle the soup into bowls and serve hot. You could garnish the soup with the black olives and red pepper flakes.

Souping

Thai Laksa Soup

Ingredients:

For the soup

- 2 packets tofu (You will need to slice the tofu into cubes of one inch each)
- 1 packet cheese slices
- 12 leaves and stalks Chinese broccoli (Often called Kai – lan. You could use regular broccoli if you want to. Make sure that you break the broccoli into smaller pieces)
- 4 carrots (You will need to peel them well and chop them into matchsticks)
- 4 zucchinis (You will need to chop them just the way you have chopped the carrots)
- 3 cucumbers (If you prefer removing the peel, you will need to remove it and then cut the cucumber into the shape of matchsticks)
- 12 tbsp. Laksa paste
- 8 cups Asian vegetable stock
- 4 cups coconut milk (Low fat)
- 4 tbsp. grated palm sugar (This is an optional ingredient)
- 2 cups coconut cream
- 3 tbsp. coconut oil

- 4 tbsp. cilantro (Chopped)
- 2 chilies (Dice them finely)
- 2 lemons (Zested and juiced)

For the Asian Vegetable Broth

- 2 medium onions (Chopped finely)
- 12 tbsp. fresh chives (Chopped)
- 4 carrots (Chopped)
- 4 celery ribs (Chopped)
- 6 cloves garlic (You will need to peel the garlic and cut the cloves finely)
- 2 sweet red peppers (Chopped finely)
- 6 tbsp. fresh ginger (You will need to peel and chop the ginger finely)
- 7 baby bok choy (These are also called Shanghai Tips. You will need to cut them into half)
- 4 stalks lemongrass (Remove the outer leaves and chop finely)
- 2 tsp. black pepper
- 2 tbsp. Kosher salt

Method:

For the Asian vegetable broth

You will need to wash all the vegetables well and prepare them. Now, place a stockpot on medium flame and add a little oil to the pot. Add the onions to the pot and sauté till they have turned golden brown and are translucent. Now, add the remaining ingredients to the pot and add the water making sure that all the vegetables are covered with the water. Add the seasoning to the pot and cover it.

Bring the stock in the pot to a boil. Now, reduce the flame and continue to simmer the ingredients in the pot. Do this after you have removed the cover from the pot. You will need to allow the broth to cool right before you drain the stock. You will need to use this broth in the soup.

For the soup

You will need to place a large saucepan over medium flame and add the coconut oil to the pan. When the oil has melted, you will need to add the laksa paste to the pan and sauté the paste for a few minutes while stirring constantly. You will need to add more of the coconut oil to the pan if you must. Now, add the stock and the lime juice to the pan and bring all the ingredients to a boil. While the ingredients are boiling, add the sugar to the pan and make sure that it has melted.

Add the tofu and the cheese slices to the pan and cook for a few minutes. Remove the tofu from the pan and place it on the cooking board. When it has cooled down, you will need to cut the tofu into smaller strips. Reduce the flame and add the coconut milk to the saucepan. Bring the ingredients in the saucepan to a simmer and add the carrots, tofu and the broccoli to the pan. You will need to add the coconut cream and stir the ingredients together. Remove the saucepan from the flame. Ladle the soup into bowls and serve it hot.

Potato Soup

Ingredients:

For the soup

- 10 large potatoes
- 6 large onions
- 4 cups butter
- 10 cups Chinese vegetable broth
- 10 stalks celery
- 15 ounces evaporated milk (Canned)
- 2 tsp. coconut oil
- Salt and pepper to taste

For the Vegetable broth

- 12 cloves garlic
- 6 cups water
- 5 – 6 carrots
- 10 potatoes
- 8 onions
- 8 celery stalks
- 3 sprigs Thyme
- 3 sprigs Rosemary
- 3 sprigs Sage
- Fresh parsley
- Sea Salt

- Pepper

Method:

For the Vegetable Stock

You will first need to chop the vegetables finely and leave them aside. Take a large stockpot and add the water to the pot. Now, add the cut vegetables to the pot and ensure that the water has covered the vegetables well. There is a possibility that you will need to add a little more water to immerse the cut vegetables fully under water. Now, add the herbs and the seasoning to the pot and mix the ingredients well together.

Place the pot on high flame and bring the water to a boil. While the water is boiling, you will need to stir the ingredient together to ensure that you obtain all the nutrients required from the vegetables. When the water has boiled for five minutes, you will need to lower the flame and let the water continue to simmer. You will need to wait till the water has become slightly thick. Taste the stock to understand if the flavor is right for you. Strain the stock from the vegetables and set it aside for the soup.

For the soup

The first thing you will need to do is peel the potatoes and cut the potatoes into cubes that are of one inch each. You will also have to chop the onions and the celery very finely. Take a saucepan and place it on medium heat. Add the oil to the pan and wait till the oil warms. Once the oil has warmed, you will need to add the onions to the pan and sauté till the onions have turned golden brown and translucent. Add the celery to the pan and continue to cook till the celery has turned brown. Now, add the potatoes to the pan and roast them well.

Add the stock to the pan and cover the lid of the pan. Cook the ingredients on medium or low flame for at least thirty minutes and wait till the ingredients boil. Once the ingredients have started to boil, reduce the heat and let the ingredients simmer. You will need to cover the pan for a few more seconds and then will need to add the milk, pepper, butter and the salt to the pan. Heat the entire soup and ladle it into the bowl. If you want the soup to be thicker, you will need to let the soup simmer for longer in the pan.

Apple Squash Soup

Ingredients:

- 4 Granny Smith apples (You will need to peel the apples and core them. Now cut the apples into quarters.)
- 2 tbsp. canola oil
- 2 cups leeks (You will need to use light green and white parts only. Make sure that you slice these parts finely)
- 3 pounds butternut squash (You will need to peel the squash and seed it. Now, cut the squash into cubes of an inch each)
- 4 cups water
- ½ cup old fashioned oats (You could use rolled oats instead)
- 3 tbsp. fresh ginger (You will need to peel and mince the ginger)
- Salt to taste
- 2 tbsp. mild curry powder

Method:

You will need to place a saucepan on medium flame and add a little oil to the pan. When the oil has heated, add the leeks to the pan and stir for a few minutes. Now, add the remaining ingredients to the pan and fry. You will need to stir the ingredients continuously. Now cover the pan and increase the flame to high. Cook the ingredients for ten minutes. Once the time is up, uncover the pan and blend the ingredients in the pan using an immersion blender. Heat the ingredients one more time and ladle the soup into the bowls.

Souping

Conclusion

In conclusion, soups are a weight loss sensation. They are very satisfying to the stomach. Soups are full of protein and vegetables. Weight loss and soups go hand in hand together. You will not leave the table feeling unsatisfied or hungry. These soup recipes are the best in the business and are just the beginning to a brand new you. Losing weight is never an easy task; however, with the proper tools you too can be successful in this new journey and life style. Soups are an essential key component of any weight loss journeys.

This isn't dieting. This is a permanent change in eating habits and life style. It's time to bring life back into your body and treat yourself right. When changing your body, your state of mind needs to be altered as well. Body and mind need to co-exist with each other in order to achieve the desires of weight loss. Never start tomorrow what you can start today. Today is your day to shine and to give you a healthier you. Let's begin today the journey with one of these recipes.

Souping

Susie Campbell

Souping

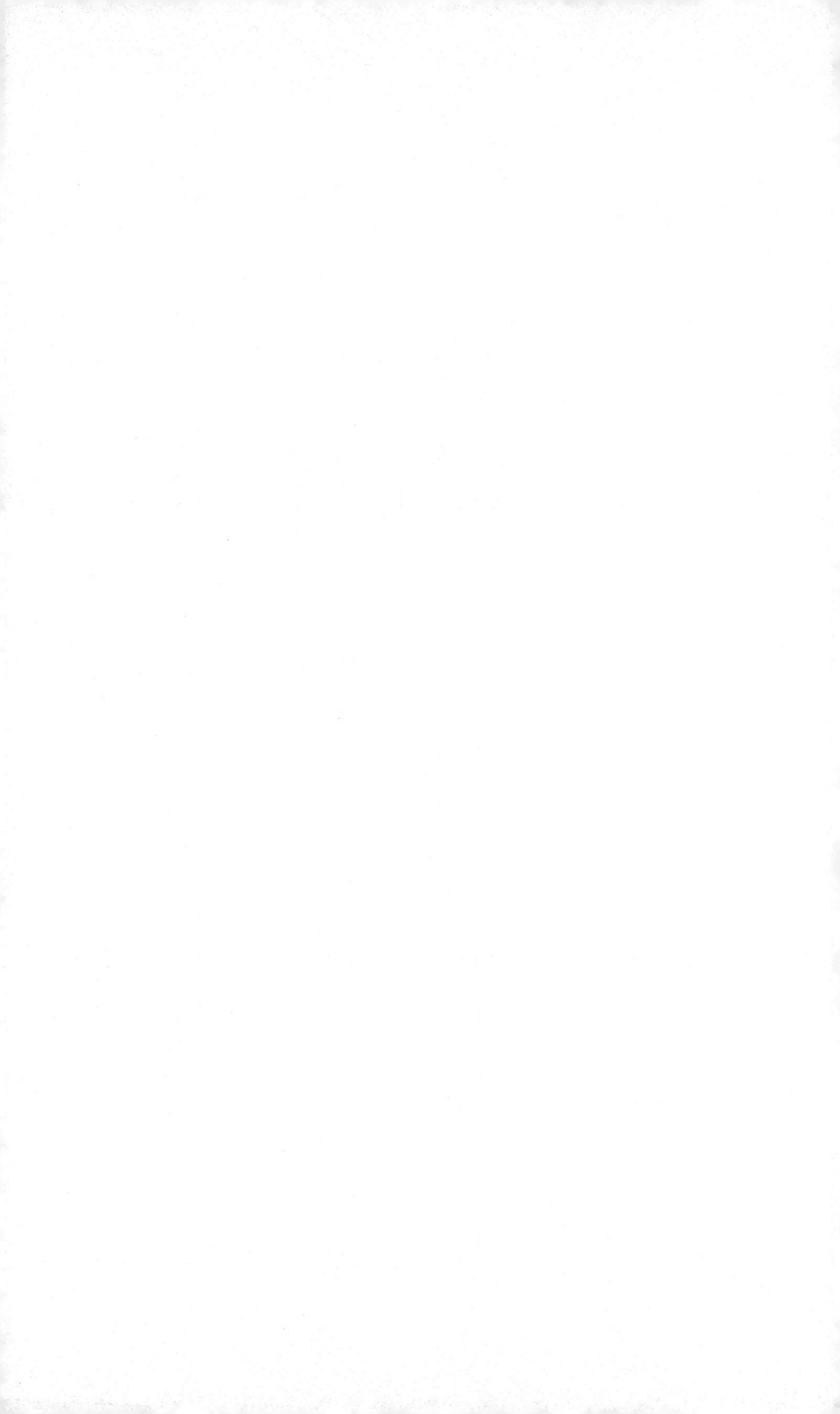

Made in the USA
Monee, IL
06 August 2023